STAYING ALIVE: MY RIDE WITH OVARIAN CANCER

ANITA GAYTON

First published 2024
by Rowanvale Books Ltd
The Gate
Keppoch Street
Roath
Cardiff
CF24 3JW
www.rowanvalebooks.com

A CIP catalogue record for this book is available from the British Library.
ISBN: 978-1-83584-033-7
Hardback ISBN: 978-1-83584-034-4
eBook ISBN: 978-1-83584-032-0

CONTENTS

BRIDGE OF HOPE

Body pressed flat
to the frost-frozen earth
focussing on the bridge ahead
hung heavy with mist in the just-breaking dawn.
Drenching damp from the icy moss melting under me
seeps through to my bones,
watery light-shafts begin to liquify the overhead icicles
to drip, drip, drip on my unprotected head.
The smell of the undergrowth mingles with the aroma
of fear,
permeating my nostrils.
It is my fear.
All reminding me of the untenability of my position.
Remaining prone is not an option.
Reminded too by my comrades behind, urging me on,
some whisper words of encouragement, one or two poke
at my ankles,
infuriating me.
I raise my head, my eyes follow the track of worn grass,
the bridge is so close, just a few steps
and I would be able to

lift my foot

onto the first plank.

It looks solid.

But then a cry, a splash, someone has gone.

Squinting into the distance I can see nothing,

just know it has happened

and it could happen to me.

I do know of others who made it to the other side

but they disappeared

into the fog, out of sight and I do not know their final destination.

What if I just start?

Just a little hope and I could reach the peak of the bridge

but maybe there is more than one peak

and I will not be strong enough

to keep going.

My face drops into the mud.

Suddenly arms take me and I am hoisted to my knees,

some crawl in front, some ease from behind,

the words in my ears whisper that I must move, I must hope

because there is no life in despair.

NOT QUITE THE BEGINNING

It was 24th September 2022 when I was asked by a doctor in A&E if I wanted to be resuscitated. Given that I had walked into the hospital myself and had been living my best life until about three months before, I replied that yes, of course I did.

'Why?' he challenged. 'Resuscitation teams are very reluctant to respond to people who are so ill.'

I was shocked, horrified and upset. There had been very little preamble to prepare me for this question. He had just told me he had looked at my notes and said to himself, *Poor lady*. He mentioned a number, but I had no idea what the number meant, except that it was, apparently, really bad.

Happily, I can confirm that I am still here. Different in many ways, but definitely still present.

So, I've decided to document what is a little over the last 18 months of my life. I'm not going to describe it as a journey, because that phrase really irritates me. As you'll see, a few things in life really irritate me. Everyone is on a journey these days. The trouble is, the end of the journey for me is probably my death—well, definitely my death, as many people have told me, and indeed I have told myself. I'm nothing special, and just like everyone else, I will die sooner or later. It's just, I really wish it wasn't this soon. Of course, I am so lucky: I am 66 years old, my sons are strong, capable men. I do not have young children to worry about. But I really wish I had longer, or that the end did not promise to be painful.

This story starts just when I was beginning to wonder if maybe there was something wrong, about March/April 2022. I thought I was just a bit constipated. I was wrong. My diagnosis of stage 4 ovarian cancer was confirmed in late August. I am still alive. It's been quite a time. I won't describe it as a roller coaster, because that is another overused and irritating phrase. I'll call it my ride with ovarian cancer. It is my story, and I am no expert in any of the issues it involves and I can't give advice, I can only talk about me. I'm hoping my story might be helpful or interesting, but we each have to find our own way with assistance from the experts.

A year or so ago, in the spring of 2022, I thought I was pretty fit and healthy. I have always been healthy, never a cold, little in the way of aches and pains, certainly no illnesses. I'd had occasional episodes of asthma since I was a child, but even that was not a problem once I realised it was a response to cats and dogs. Funny thing is, I was always worried that I would suffer from dementia as I got older. I have worked with people with dementia for many years and really didn't want to end up that way. So, when I retired I became a Dementia Friend, giving talks about dementia. I spent my time in other gainful pursuits, trying to learn new things—one of the best ways of staving off cognitive decline. I took up some studying with the Open University, completed the daily newspaper puzzles. I even tried, unsuccessfully, to learn to ride a motorbike. Well, I bought the bike and had lessons, managing, just, to pass the CBT test (compulsory basic training, not cognitive behavioural therapy as I thought) to allow me to ride on the road. I imagined myself donning my leathers in my retirement, travelling around Europe, having adventures. I gave up the motorbike dream fairly early. It was when a pedal cyclist overtook me on a corner that I realised perhaps I hadn't got that daredevil, throw-caution-to-the-wind attitude required. I ponder now whether being killed suddenly on a motorbike would be better than a slow death from cancer? I suppose the thing is, you just can't choose. Probably a good thing really, as you'd be bound to change your mind halfway through. So, I'm on a different ride now, just as scary, with many uphill climbs, not knowing what's around the corner, and a destination I don't want to reach. However, I am still enjoying riding along.

In May 2022, things were generally pretty good. That month we'd had a big family and friends party in a local village hall to make up for all the celebrations we'd missed during Covid. I'd played in a walking football tournament. I had wanted to play football since childhood but girls' teams weren't allowed at that time, so I was pretty chuffed that at last I had achieved my ambition. I'd been to the Hay Literary Festival, pitched my tent and walked the mile or so to the venue each day. Life was very good. However, I thought my fitness had deteriorated.

I've never been super fit, just liked taking part in things. I've done a couple of marathons, 15 or more years ago, but my times were over five and a half hours, so it was just a gentle jog, with quite a lot of walking at the end. During the first Covid lockdown, I downloaded a running app and started on 'Couch to 5k'. Like many people, I decided I would make the most of the enforced isolation. I completed the programme and felt I was on the up again.

Then it was the second lockdown and I just never improved. Any slight upward gradient could have been a mountain, I got so puffed out. *OK,* I thought, *I just need to try harder*, and with a bit of persuasion from a friend, joined a running group. I was quite nervous about it, but they were very welcoming of beginners and I managed the running exercises really well. However, it was the journey there and back that was the problem. The group met about a mile away from my home, so I walked to the park where it was held. That was when I noticed that I really needed the toilet when I arrived, having to nip into the nearby pub. Same problem again when I was on my way home. It was literally a close-run thing to get back unsullied. *Hmm,* I thought. *Perhaps I need to change my diet to get my bowels back to more predictable workings.* Then I found the lump in my abdomen. I have never really trusted myself, so I wondered if I had always had a lump there and just not noticed it. *Oh right, must be constipation causing a blockage,* I thought. I'm not sure now why I was so confident in my medical diagnostic abilities. I called the GP surgery. No appointments that week, and the diary wasn't made up for the following week. Well, I was going away for a few days and it would probably resolve itself during that time. A nagging doubt told me it might be serious, but I dismissed it. I felt so well, other than a bit of a bowel problem.

I saw the GP in June. She examined me and I saw the look on her face. That's when I really knew it was serious.

'Have you lost weight?' she asked.

'Ha ha ha, I wish,' I replied stupidly, as though this were all a joke.

She gave me a pitying look. 'I'll fast-track you on the cancer pathway,' she said, 'but that doesn't mean it is cancer.' She was clearly not a woman who played poker, as her face shouted otherwise.

Even so, I went home and googled every other possibility and even slightly convinced myself that it could be some of them. I mean, I felt so healthy.

THE NIGHTMARE FIRST FEW MONTHS

Once I actually got into the system in mid-September, I received good service from the NHS. July and August, however, were like a waking nightmare. I know now that I should have gone to the GP a few months earlier, at the first sign of the bowel change. I did not realise that cancer would cause me to crash from feeling really healthy to feeling completely debilitated within weeks. I was foolish to wait.

I have always religiously complied with all screenings: smear tests, mammograms and bowel screenings—but have also always had confidence that my body wouldn't let me down. So, having said I won't give advice, I'm now going to offer some. I would urge everyone not to make the same mistake as me. As they say in all the warnings, if you notice a change in your bowel habits, see your GP straightaway. I know it's not easy. Even now the thought of hanging on the phone at 8 a.m. every morning to be told to phone back at 8 a.m. the next day gives a feeling of gloom. But if you don't bother, the outcome might be a lot more gloomy.

While I blamed myself for not seeking help straightaway, the speed at which I then received tests and appointments did not seem fast enough, and it was only thanks to pushing by me, family and friends that I started to get the treatment I needed. Nothing would happen unless I chased it, and I didn't even know who or what to chase. The promises around the fast-track cancer pathway initially gave a bit of confidence. I was pleased when it began within a few days with a phone call from a colorectal nurse specialist who asked lots of questions and referred me for a colonoscopy. I wonder now if I had actually had a face-to-face appointment where I was examined by a doctor whether I would have been identified as having ovarian cancer rather than going down the bowel cancer route, which might have saved a bit of time.

The colonoscopy was not pleasant, particularly the concoction you have to drink to clear out the bowel the day before. It started off OK, and I wondered why I had heard people complain about it. After several more glassfuls over the next few hours, I felt like Dumbledore drinking from the Horcrux vessel and only wished Harry Potter was with me to help force it down. Sorry, any non-Potter fans to whom that won't make sense. Anyway, I must have done OK with it, because the colonoscopy report noted that 'bowel preparation was excellent'. I felt strangely proud.

Apart from the triumph of my magnificent bowel preparation, the rest of the colonoscopy was not successful and could not be fully completed. It appeared there was a 'proximal sigmoid' obstruction. Well, those were some of the words, hopefully in the right order, which I was told meant there was something pressing on the bowel from the outside rather than the obstruction being in the bowel. The bowel consultant told me that because of the lack of result from the colonoscopy, I needed a special scan colonoscopy. As these were specialist procedures, there was about a six- to eight-week wait. I didn't think I had that long. I spent a day phoning around private facilities to see if I could get one somewhere else more quickly. The answer appeared to be no. I might have been able to get an appointment with a private consultant in a couple of weeks, but that was just for an initial assessment, not the procedure itself. I was in despair, getting increasingly frightened and panicky.

My niece, Sally, suggested I contact the bowel consultant's secretary and ask to speak to him again. I had not realised that the secretary was a major player and a key route to the consultant. The secretary organised for the consultant to call me, and a different plan was organised. I would have other scans and biopsies and be passed to the gynaecology team. In NHS terms, the investigations were probably arranged quickly, a week between everything. The problem for me was that I was deteriorating at speed. My bowels were not working properly, and I could not move far from a toilet. My breathing was getting worse—because of fluid around the lung, I was told. How had that happened? Where does it come from?

By the end of July, so only two months on from when I had felt fine, I was seriously debilitated. My tickets to the Commonwealth Games opening ceremony were passed on to my niece. I was too unwell to walk more than a few steps. I was still waiting to see the gynaecology consultant. Apparently, I had to be discussed in the weekly multi-disciplinary team meeting before any progress could be made. They only discussed two new patients a week. Unfortunately for me, and probably several others, the consultant was on holiday. I was rescheduled. The consultant caught Covid. I was rescheduled.

During this time, I had been referred to the chest clinic because my breathing was so bad. The referral seemed to have got lost. In desperation, when I was in the hospital for a blood test, I found my way into the chest clinic without an appointment. It was quite a walk from the car park to the clinic. Due to Covid requirements and my own vulnerability, I was wearing a mask, and I was gasping for breath by the time I reached the waiting room. At reception, I enquired if they had my referral. I could barely get the words out. They didn't think they had. I said I needed an appointment. The clinics were full for the following week, I was told. If I went away, they said, they would try and find out what had happened with my referral and let me know. I was not going to be fobbed off that easily. I was determined I was not going to leave the hospital that day without something being arranged. I was in tears by this time, my mask being sucked into my mouth with every inhalation. I said I would go for my blood test but was going to come back. When I returned, I was even more breathless and told to take a seat. Eventually, I was told I could come back the following Monday if I was prepared to wait to be seen. I certainly was. It felt like a minor triumph—as long as I lasted till then. While that might sound overdramatic, it really isn't. I tend to underplay rather than overplay. At the rate things were going downhill, I thought I hadn't got long left.

I lasted the week and managed to be seen at the chest clinic. One of the surprises from this consultation was that the respiratory consultant was the first to really confirm the cancer diagnosis. Until that point, medics had said things like 'sinister' and 'mass'. The doctor probably thought I knew already, so there was no warm-up to the word 'cancer'.

They identified fluid around my lung and recommended a pleural tap. I thought this was a pop group, but no, it's when a needle is inserted into your back, which then draws off fluid through a tube into a big bag. I was quite terrified at this prospect. I thought that the needle would go into my lungs and if it went wrong that my lung would be punctured and I would whizz round the clinic, making raspberry noises like a deflating balloon. I was wrong about all of that. It seems to be a pretty routine procedure, as evidenced by the response I received when I asked the two very young doctors if they had done this before. Apparently they had, many times. The fluid would be drawn off from around my lungs to ease my breathing and also so that some could be sent for analysis.

My elder son, Will, came with me. It was not anywhere near as bad as I'd feared. Well, nothing probably could have been, as I had built it up into something quite horrendous. The needle does not go into your lungs; the fluid is in a pleural cavity at the side of the lungs, so whizzing around the room is unlikely. It was also relatively painless by the time the local anaesthetic had got to work. Once it was underway, it was even quite interesting to see the pink fluid draining into bags. It also made breathing quite a bit easier, so a fairly fundamental requirement achieved.

July and August saw more investigations, scans and an ultrasound-guided biopsy. I still hadn't seen the gynaecological oncologist. I had, however, been allocated a clinical nurse specialist (CNS), and what a great support she was. She would report back to me results and any progress or otherwise towards starting treatment, and I always felt she was on my side. She told me that a bowel obstruction was extremely serious and must be avoided at all costs. This meant cutting out as much fibre from my diet as possible. In other words: look at a healthy diet sheet and then remove anything healthy. My meals were now completely white. I felt my life was reduced to basics. I realised that, for the immediate future, my job was to make sure I breathed, ate, drank and pooed. Anything else was a bonus. I even kept daily records. Not the breathing, obviously. I thought that if I was recording the other three then the breathing could be taken as read.

The other surprise around this time was that, as well as my pleural cavities filling up with fluid, my abdomen was too. I'm not kidding, I looked 13-months pregnant. My clothes no longer fitted me, and I looked like the proverbial beached whale. My elder son took me to a charity shop to see if they had any maternity clothes as I didn't want to waste money on garments which, for good or ill, I wasn't going to wear for long. He asked an assistant if they had any maternity dresses and pointed at me. To be fair, the woman managed not to look too confused and/or horrified as to how this old woman could have got pregnant—and with such a good-looking young man.

The CNS arranged for me to be booked into the hospital to drain off some of the abdominal fluid. It took all day, and I was attached to a succession of bags to collect the fluid. While it helped a bit, I was hoping for a more dramatic improvement, not to find that only one of the triplets had been delivered. Looks like I needn't have ordered the crop top.

The third week of August saw our annual big family holiday in Shropshire; as usual, there were about 20 of us. It was wonderful but poignant. We have been doing this for many years, and I was pretty sure this would be my last. A lot of others on the holiday thought so too. My niece brought a SATS machine with her to keep an eye on my oxygen saturation levels. I was exempt from my turn cooking the dinner—there has to be some bonus for playing the cancer card.

It was during that week that my CNS phoned as she had promised she would if I was discussed at last by the multi-disciplinary team. I took my phone and sat at one of the picnic benches in the holiday home garden, with a beautiful view over the Shropshire hills. I was prepared with my pen and notebook to note whatever she might tell me. I wrote 'Stage 4a ovarian cancer'. Most women, she said, only present at this late stage because there are few warning signs. She also explained that they call cancers by where they first appear, and mine had spread to a number of different organs. I wrote steadily, keen to record her words accurately. By doing that, I could distance myself, as though I was taking lecture notes for a future exam. She said I had been discussed and the consultant was going to take me on. I had an appointment in two weeks' time.

The world stood still for a moment. I recognised what a tough job she had and thanked her for her call. I hung up. Then realisation smacked me in the head and I cried angrily. Fortunately it was a remote cottage, as the profusion of fucks I sobbed through clenched teeth and clenched fists would have had the place closed down. My lovely sister and niece were keeping an eye on me and were there to comfort me. They had their work cut out, because there is no comfort. No words can make it better. Hugs and physical touch are the only solace. I eventually pulled myself together and went into our lovely holiday home to seek out my sons to tell them the diagnosis had been confirmed. By this time, this was no surprise for any of us. I guess, though, that we had all hoped that somehow it would not be as bad as we feared. I hated telling them. I hated causing them pain. They were fabulous, too, more hugs and a very measured response.

Back from the holiday, my oncology appointment was postponed again, for another two weeks. The consultant had to catch up on all the other patients he had missed while he had Covid. Then he had study leave booked. I found his private secretary's number to try and book a private appointment, even though I didn't have health insurance. She said she would try and help. She did and the appointment was moved back to its original date. There is obviously nothing untoward about a medic having a holiday or being ill—I also want my consultant to be at the top of her or his game and continuing to learn.

But surely there should be enough slack in the system for this to be manageable without putting lives at risk.

It was a long two weeks, and in the meantime I planned to go away for the weekend to attend my elder son, Will's, book launch in Cardiff. Nothing was going to keep me away from that if it was the last thing I did. By the Sunday, I wondered if that might actually be the case. The morning we were due to travel home, I felt terrible, my breathing unreliable. I measured my oxygen levels, as I now had my own little machine. It read 82. I googled that and it said to go to hospital immediately. I had a choice to make. I felt the sensible thing to do would be to go to the accident and emergency in Cardiff, but I really didn't want to go to a hospital so far away from home. I just wanted to get home. Fortunately, I wasn't driving so I sat in the passenger seat, trying to breathe deeply in front of the air vents. I realised I needed help urgently. At last we were approaching my hometown, but I knew I couldn't get all the way to my house. I asked to be dropped off at my local accident and emergency department.

I could barely walk into A&E. I could see there was a queue under a veranda-like structure outside. It's not like me to queue-jump, but this once I made an exception. Fortunately, a paramedic waiting by her ambulance saw I was not in a good way. She took me inside to where they were booking in arrivals. I explained about the cancer and the difficulty breathing and had a magnificent response. They quickly got me to a chair inside and started me on oxygen. What a relief. Oxygen is delicious. Never underestimate the value of breathing.

I have already described some of the ensuing resuscitation conversation that completely floored me. The junior doctor accompanying the consultant who had questioned my desire to live realised that I was very upset. She kindly stayed back while he moved on, and asked me if I had any questions. Then she said, 'The main thing is to have faith.' My distress turned to fury. Inside my head I replied, *No, it fucking isn't. The main thing is to get some treatment.* But my mouth said, 'I don't have any questions, thank you.' Her comment might have been helpful for some people but not for me. It seemed like she was saying I was about to die, that nothing could prevent it and I could only look forward to the afterlife, not this one. For someone who doesn't believe in an afterlife, that was pretty bleak.

IN HOSPITAL AT LAST

In A&E, they discovered clots in my lungs. Another surprise and another test of my clearly inadequate medical knowledge. I had thought my breathing problems were the result of the fluid build-up, but this was a pulmonary embolism. Cancer, it seems, can do whatever it likes to your body. The decision was made for me to be admitted. I was so relieved that at last I would receive some treatment. Unfortunately, there was no free bed on the oncology ward.

My outpatient appointment was due with the consultant, and I assumed that he would come to see me on the ward. I was informed that he didn't see inpatients. I replied that, in that case, I would discharge myself. Eventually, with much communication, helped by my family, friends and the clinical nurse specialist, the consultant visited me on the ward. Lucky he did, as my son Will had stationed himself on the ward and was determined he was not going to leave until I had been seen.

It was a very helpful meeting. Everything was laid out on the table in all its stark detail. At last, I knew my options, agreed to treatment and we could get started. We asked how long I might have. This is going to sound very strange, but I had forgotten what the doctor said until I was talking to Will about it recently. Apparently he said two years. I don't know how I could have forgotten that. Nearly two years on, it seems a very short time, but when I was told that, it seemed unbelievable that I could last that long.

Anyway, four days after being admitted and a couple of ward moves later, a space came up on the oncology ward. It was such a relief to have reached the right place. I was pretty sure, however, that it was the very same room that my dad had been in before he died of leukaemia. Anyway, time for chemotherapy.

CHEMOTHERAPY: WHAT'S YOUR POISON?

Everyone has heard of chemotherapy and knows it's not a nice thing. Everyone who receives it is very different, and patients receive different drugs in different dosages on different schedules, so I can't tell you what side-effects anyone will have from chemo. I can only describe what it has been like for me.

My first session took place in the hospital ward as, following my emergency admission, I was still an inpatient and my condition meant that I needed to be closely monitored. Because I was so ill, I was only given one of the two intended drugs, and a nurse sat with me as it was entering my veins. It's a bit hard to know at this point whether the symptoms I experienced were a result of the cancer or the chemo. Nothing much happened for the first 24 hours, and then I just felt like death. The nausea was overwhelming and I could do very little other than lie on the bed. I remember thinking that if this was my new life then I didn't want it. I felt terrible for my visitors because I found it difficult to converse. This was not like me.

I did not know how the chemo would affect me or for how long. I just lay on the bed in despair. I could not eat. Meals were put in front of me but I could not face them. The ward domestic assistant recognised how terrible I felt and asked if I would like a rich tea biscuit. At the time it felt like the kindest thing anyone had ever done for me. It was just what I needed, and I managed to eat the biscuit.

There is medication you can take for the nausea, and stronger drugs if required. They helped a bit, but only time seemed to really make a difference. After a week, I started to feel a bit better and the side-effects began to reduce. I was able to go home. The only blot on the horizon was that a new round of chemo would come every three weeks. Just as you are on the up, you get whacked back down again.

Before you start chemotherapy, you are given a leaflet—well, more of a booklet—about the side-effects that might be expected. It does not make for happy reading. I don't know if anyone gets all of them, but I certainly achieved quite a selection. Each round of chemo followed pretty much the same pattern. The first day or so afterwards I felt not too bad. At that point, it's easy to think that you are doing really well. Day two, and the nausea got steadily worse, as well as intense exhaustion. I wonder too if they put misery fluid in those little bags of chemo medication? They pump it in and it sits around for a couple of days until, whoosh, the droplets of 'life isn't worth living if it's going to be this shit' start travelling round your veins. Some comes out through your eye sockets, which helps a bit, but the rest gets to your brain, worms its way round and throws into your consciousness every shit thing about this situation.

I also had a terrible rash that was apparently contact dermatitis. Itching everywhere clothes touched me was really unpleasant. I was tempted to walk around stark naked but realised that, as I would have to sit down at some point and therefore touch the chair, this wasn't the perfect solution. And, of course, it wasn't my best look. Antihistamines and liberal use of calamine lotion turned out to be the better option. I hadn't had calamine lotion lathered on me since I was a child with sunburn. (Don't blame my parents—those were the days when sunburn was fine.) I'd forgotten how it leaves you with a white sheen. If I'd looked near death before, once the calamine was on I was definitely on the verge.

Some side-effects diminish but others do not always go away. Again, this varies for different people, but for me the peripheral neuropathy, a tingling and numbness in your extremities, i.e. toes and fingers, has improved but is still there. Initially, things like taking the top off the shower gel were annoyingly difficult. There isn't always someone readily available to pop their head in the shower and help with that one. It's not a major problem at the moment, but it still feels a bit weird when you can't feel some of your toes.

One surprise has been hearing loss. Prior to the treatment, I'd thought that my hearing wasn't as good as it used to be and put it down to increasing age. Halfway through my chemo rounds, however, I noticed quite a radical deterioration. I asked the oncologist about it, could it be related? He put up his hands and said, 'Guilty as charged.' Oh well. Next stop, the GP for a referral to audiology.

One of the many challenges with chemotherapy is that it makes you vulnerable to infections. At the end of a chemo session, you are sent home with injections to boost your white blood cells. When I was due for discharge from hospital after my first chemo, I was horrified to be given injections to take home with me. 'But I can't do that,' I said to the nurse. 'There's no way I can inject myself.' She asked me if there was anyone else at home who could do it. No, there wasn't.

I was thinking fast. Could I go to the GP surgery and have a nurse do it? No, they don't do that. Could I stay with my niece who is a nurse, who lives 70 miles away? No, of course I couldn't. Reluctantly, I accepted the situation and the nurse showed me how to do it myself. I asked her to write down the instructions because, although it is very straightforward, I was in such a state of panic that I thought I would forget. I'm not quite sure how it's even possible to get it wrong, but I wanted to cover all angles, literally. It turned out that I could do it, and it was the least of my problems.

As you are immunocompromised, at least for part of the time between rounds of chemo, it is important to avoid situations where there is a greater risk of infection. This is sometimes quite hard to explain to people, particularly those who want to hug you. I've never been a particularly huggy person, especially with people I'd only consider acquaintances, but people often tried to hug me without warning. I know they just wanted to show support, but it can be a bit scary when you are trying to avoid catching something.

My attempts to avoid contamination were confounded by the family Christmas. A couple of days later, I wasn't feeling too brilliant and had a slight temperature. Elder son was insistent that I call the emergency assessment bay at the hospital. I, of course, still not having learned the lesson of asking for help quickly, was reluctant.

The emergency bay is a great thing, available to any oncology patient with a health concern. You can call any time of the day or night for advice. I looked at my cancer treatment book, and raised temperature was on the red list. I called and they said to come in. I was sure I would only be there briefly. They did various tests, and not long afterwards called me into a side room and told me I had Covid. At that time, the service for vulnerable people like me with Covid was excellent, although few people in the hospital or the GP surgery seemed to know how it all worked. I searched for the email I had received from the NHS a few months before and reported my positive test on the system. By early the next day, I had been contacted and was in receipt of antivirals. They must have been effective because I recovered much more quickly than other members of my family.

So, chemotherapy is pretty rough. I had six rounds by the end of 2022, the last one on 23rd December. I had two further ones whilst I was recovering from my surgery. Those last two felt like being kicked while I was down.

I wonder why they call them 'rounds' of chemotherapy instead of 'sessions' or 'treatments'. I've decided it's because they are more like rounds in boxing. You keep getting hit, and hopefully you stand back up again. Thankfully, I didn't have all the possible side-effects, but I had enough. It reminded me of earlier in my career when I worked with people addicted to alcohol. The toxic effects of chemo had the same results as those of chronic alcoholism. I just wished I could have started off with the fun bit.

Apart from the first one, all my rounds were in the chemo suite at the hospital. The staff in there are lovely and kind. You have to go prepared, however: books, puzzles, drinks, food, snacks. I am always relieved when the canula is in, as it seems to be getting harder to find a vein. I'm always told I have very short veins, which clearly makes no sense. They must go somewhere. What they really mean apparently is that mine go round corners, so finding one that is long enough to get the whole needle in is tricky. The other frustrations are the time it takes for the drugs to arrive from the pharmacy, sometimes hours, and that any slight adverse movement of the hand with the canula in causes the flow to stop. Sometimes every patient's machine seems to be beeping at the same time, with nurses rushing around getting them going again.

The thing that's important to remember with chemo is that while the first week is dreadful, the second and third week gradually improve. Sometimes it's very hard to remember that though.

I haven't had chemo for several months now, although I still go in to the chemo suite every three weeks for 'infusions'. More on that later. It is very likely, however, that I will have more chemo in the future if, or when, the cancer re-emerges. It's powerful stuff and we were told 'it had done its job' in that it made removal of the cancer possible in my surgery. So, a necessary evil.

HAIR TODAY, GONE QUITE QUICKLY

Hair is quite a big thing in cancer—well, to be more precise, chemotherapy. Some drugs make you lose your hair and some don't. It's one of the first things the CNS asks you: 'How do you feel about losing your hair?' Apparently that influences their choice of drug. I know losing your hair is devastating for some people. It wasn't really that big a deal for me. I mean, don't get me wrong, I'd rather have hair. But it was never my crowning glory. I've tried different styles all my life and was never that thrilled with any of them. I asked my elder son once—he was an adult by this time—'Why does my hair never suit me?'

After some consideration he said, quite brutally, 'Perhaps it's your face?'

I realised he was right and from then on had my hair however I wanted it. So, having no hair was not too much of a worry for me. *Better to be bald*, I thought, *than have flowing locks in your coffin*.

You can have a cold cap whilst having your chemo session, which may help your hair stay attached to your scalp. I did a bit of research—well, googling—on that one. It looked as though it made your session longer, could be painful and was not always successful. So, not for me. And to be honest, I was quite intrigued by the hair loss thing, how it happened, when and what I would look like. The answer to the last one, by the way, is that I looked like a member of Britain First hoping for a fight.

Nothing happened after the first chemo session. Hair still all in place, me feeling pretty cocky. Then I found out that because I had been so ill—that was underselling it, I'd had a near-death experience—they had only given me one of the two prescribed drugs as the medics didn't think my body could cope with them both. I'd received the one that didn't cause hair loss. Less cocky now.

The situation changed after subsequent sessions. The main learning point is that hair loss is such a nuisance. How much hair can one person have? Everyone was very lovely. The beauty person at the hospital fitted me up with a wig that looked remarkably like my hair. People gave me hats and scarves, and my wonderful niece even offered to do a joint head shave together. I refused, as Sally has lovely hair and it would have been a waste. I had my hair cut short instead, but I can tell you, that still leaves an awful lot of hair to find in the bed, the bath, the shower, the kitchen and in all of the hats. I had to buy a plug-hole catcher to prevent it from blocking the drains. In the end, I put my head over the bath and pulled most of it out while my partner aimed the shower at my head. It still left more than you'd think, but it was a relief not to have to vacuum the bed every day.

I can't really offer advice on headwear. All I can say is that I felt lucky it was winter. I've always been more of a bobble hat/outdoor gear sort of person than a fashion hat wearer. So, beanie hats it was, in the main. When I wanted to dress up, I tended to go for the pretty scarf/turban-type headwear, and friends would say how lovely it looked. Not to me. I looked like a woman with cancer because that's the usual headgear. My hair has grown a bit now, and I was rather pleased with it initially. I thought I looked quite edgy and decided that I have a nice skull. What a bonus from all of this. People say your hair grows back differently after chemo. The chemo curl, apparently.

I was hoping for blonde curls to appear. But no, just a tight, 80s-style perm, and still the same face.

Eyebrows disappear too, and you would not believe how weird that looks. Sally suggested eyebrow tattoos. I have always been ideologically opposed to tattoos—it's my age—so couldn't really contemplate it. But could you imagine if you had tattooed eyebrows and then your real ones grew back but in a slightly different position? Double-decker eyebrows.

I must also mention the non-head hair. Yes, you know what I'm talking about, the hair you never wanted in the first place. Another bonus. What a saving on time and/or beauty therapists. Then it grows back. Never before have I had nose hair. Now I have to pluck it. As a double whammy, it makes me sneeze. Because of my stoma, I have to wear a support belt (I call it my Liz Truss) when nose plucking in order to prevent a hernia. Legs and lady bits have to be trimmed. Not only that, but they have developed an extra bushiness. Trust me to get the chemo curl down there.

It will soon be time to book my first hairdresser's appointment in nine months. It's now stopped being edgy, it's just curly. A friend said I looked as though I was wearing one of those old-fashioned swimming hats that had plastic flowers sticking out all over them. I'll have to think about what to chat to the hairdresser about, because it won't be holidays.

AUTUMN DAYS

So, after my discharge in early September, I continued to exist, wondering whether I would see Christmas. That whole period feels a bit of a blur. It was a heady mix of anger, frustration, nausea and weakness. I also knew I was very lucky because of the amount of support I had. My amazing sister Yvonne rearranged her life to be with me after every round of chemo. Everyone was really careful about where they went and who they mixed with to avoid me catching something when my immunity was most compromised.

During that time, my chest was not improving and the chest clinic doctor suggested a couple of alternatives to prevent build-up of fluid around my pleural cavity. This was to avoid having to go in regularly for the fluid to be drained off. The one I plumped for was to have an indwelling catheter. This meant that there was a tube fitted into my back so the fluid could be drained off by a district nurse, as required. Once again, I was terrified, and once again, the staff were amazing. The nurse was teaching a doctor how to do the procedure so I got the full rundown of what was going on behind my back. Strangely, I quite like this and can get distracted by how interesting it all is. And again, once the anaesthetic has gone in, the pain is mainly dealt with.

It felt very strange to have a tap on my back, and I had wondered if I'd have to pop down to B&Q and choose my own faucet. Happily not, and I was surprised by how inconspicuous the tap was. It didn't affect my daily activities, other than waiting in for the district nurse. After a few weeks, there was little draining out, and it was assumed the chemo had dried up the fluid. I was able to return to the hospital and have it all removed, again with very little discomfort. My breathing still isn't great, but I don't believe I'm drowning in fluid at this point.

In December, I started having some strange twinges in my chest, generally in the centre. These frightened me but they were quite fleeting. While thinking that perhaps I was having a heart attack, I still hadn't learned the lesson about going for help and did not do anything about it immediately. Well, the twinges disappeared as soon as they came. After a couple of weeks, I decided that if I had them again I would contact the emergency assessment bay, which is what I did. I was hoping they would ask me to come in, do a quick ECG and all would be fine. Unfortunately, they said to go to A&E.

It was a Saturday just before Christmas and A&E was packed to the gunnels. I was triaged fairly quickly and the staff were concerned about my vulnerability to infection given that I was mid-chemo. However, there was no spare room that I could be isolated in. I went to the waiting room, where we were squashed in like sardines. I felt that my risk of a heart attack was less than my risk of infection, so I told the staff I would walk around outside until it was my turn. So that's what I did for several hours. It was too cold to sit anywhere for long, and I would pop back to A&E every half hour to see if it was my turn yet. They had my mobile phone number and I was told they would call me, but given the number of patients, I wasn't sure that message would have been passed on.

I was right, and after about four hours when I went back in to check, I was met by a doctor who had been trying to find me and was a little irritated that I had disappeared. It all moved fairly quickly then, and after an hour or so I'd had the ECG, which appeared to be fine. I was sent to another waiting room and sat there for a while. Eventually, I asked if there was anything else and could I be on my way. I think they had forgotten me—not surprising with the avalanche of people they had been dealing with.

A week later, I had a telephone check-up with the chest-pain doctor, and six months later, an echocardiogram. Nothing untoward was found, other than the fluid around my lungs. I was pretty chuffed that I could tick off my heart as one of the organs I needn't worry about.

Apart from the nausea and weakness, the main challenge throughout this time was chasing things again. I needed drainage bags and dressing packs for the nurses who came nearly every day to drain my catheter. I was told I would need to get these via the surgery. Everything I tried in order to communicate this requirement was unsuccessful. I went into the surgery, I put notes in the prescription box, I tried to order them online. Nothing worked.

There was a similar problem with a prescription for medication. Never having been ill before, I thought that when my discharge letter from the hospital to the GP said I would need certain drugs, that those drugs would be put onto a prescription. Or if the hospital consultant said 'change this drug from an injection to oral meds' that it would happen. I won't make that mistake again. Nothing seems to happen unless the patient makes it happen. It felt such a slog, at a time when I was at my most depleted in energy. I still don't know what the problem is, but in future I might resort back to the tactic of 'I'm not moving out of here until this is sorted'. I don't really want to, though. I know most staff are trying really hard, but there does seem to be a problem with creating a smooth system.

Anyway, enough moaning. I was still alive, thanks to the NHS, and I was edging my way towards Christmas! One I'd never thought I would see. I sent my Christmas cards early, just in case. I wrote a poem for each person who would be at the Christmas dinner and put each inside a bauble. I didn't want them to forget me when I wasn't there for the following Christmas.

However, in the weeks before the next chemo round, I'd gradually started feeling better. Just the operation to get through now, and more rounds of chemotherapy.

DEBULKING

It's a great word, isn't it. Sounds so positive. It's the term they give to the surgical procedure to get rid of as much of the cancer as possible. I like to think of it more as a decluttering, having a bit of a clear out of the stuff you no longer need. That's an optimistic way of describing it. I no longer need my ovaries, womb and fallopian tubes. I can't imagine how it must be for women of child-bearing age who have to come to terms with so much physical loss, as well as the loss of dreams and future plans. The surgeons also removed quite a bit else of mine, too: lymph nodes, gall bladder, omentum. I didn't know I had an omentum before that. It's apparently the layer of fat located inside the abdomen. If I'd known that before, I could have blamed my omentum for making me look fat. Anyway, that and other organs were removed. I can't remember exactly what they told me had gone. I even had to go to a hospital out of my area where they apparently have expertise in diaphragmatic stripping. Who's ever heard of that? If it had passed my consciousness, I would have presumed it was something you did to a car, perhaps when your big end had gone.

The surgery was a big deal. The handout I was given was entitled 'Ultra-radical (extensive) surgery for advanced intra-abdominal gynaecological cancer'. Clearly one adjective was not enough to emphasise its seriousness.

There is no breaking it gently. No medic minced their words when it came to telling me about risk factors, and boy, there were a lot of risks. The pre-med with the anaesthetist and the consultation with the surgeon were pretty much all about the risks. Too many to remember, except that I was told that I would not be the same again. That felt like quite a big thing. Even if I recovered well, I was going to be a different me afterwards, and there was no going back.

They were right. My body is different now. A scar runs from between my breasts to my pubic bone. It seems a shame it's not a zip in case they need to do a bit more in the future. I have a bag permanently attached to my abdomen. I can't run anymore or walk up the stairs without it being a strain on my lungs. But I am still here. My life is still enjoyable.

I had a number of worries before the surgery. One was that I would not survive it, just die on the operating table. I suddenly realised my will was out of date, so I saw a solicitor and redid it in the week prior to the surgery. Death, however, wasn't my number one concern. Having a stroke was a bigger worry. I could not bear the thought of being paralysed or not able to speak, or trying to speak but not being understood. The other anxiety was that they might not carry out the operation at all. I was told they would open me up and have a good look round. If they felt that any organ was irredeemably damaged and the outcome would not be good then they would sew me back up again. This felt a terrible prospect. All that surgery, to be told on waking up that you were a lost cause. My family were relieved when I was in surgery for so many hours—the surgeons must have felt I was worth it.

Risk factors and probabilities are a strange thing because they do not really help decision-making in the slightest. When I was pregnant with my younger son, a blood test indicated I had a 1-in-35 chance of the baby having Down's syndrome. But you don't know if you are on the 1 side or the 34.

This time, the doctor told me a lot of numbers associated with the various risks. He asked if I would like to see the bar chart of how I compared with the average American. I agreed, as I'm a bit of a sucker for a nice graph, and it was very interesting and slightly reassuring. When you are talking about numbers it's so much easier, makes it seem more objective and easier to talk about, until you remember it's about you. Risk of death was 1–2%, so the bars on the bar chart didn't look too high, but it was all still a little bit meaningless.

The information handout was not entirely reassuring. It answered the question I had asked the anaesthetist: 'What if I don't have the surgery?' He said it was a good question. Having always been a bit of a good girl swot, I was rather pleased, although in reality it was my niece who had suggested I ask that question. The information handout said that five-year survival rates for women with advanced ovarian cancer who had the radical surgery were between 31% and 47% compared with 14% to 35% in patients who had standard surgery. The median survival rate for women having the ultra-radical surgery was 50 months. Whichever way you look at the numbers, it wasn't great, but it suggested I would have a better chance of living a little bit longer if I had the radical surgery. So, I signed the consent form. The copy of the letter from the anaesthetist said that I was 'at an increased risk of complications but likely to survive'. It wasn't a great vote of confidence but you've got to take what you're given.

The team at the Royal Derby Hospital were brilliant. I remember saying to my sister, who accompanied me to every appointment, that I felt as though I were a private patient. I was talked to as though we were a collaborative team, that my views were important, that

I needed all the information, however unpalatable. I seemed to be really important to them. I know this should be standard, but I can't tell you how grateful I was. I felt so vulnerable, so scared, and these 'soft skills', often underrated, gave me confidence in them and in myself. An example of their flexibility was that, as I lived so far away, they arranged for me to be admitted the day before my surgery for a blood transfusion rather than make an additional journey during the week. This made so much difference.

At my pre-op appointment, I also saw the physiotherapist. I was given a little machine called a spirometer which I had to take home and practise with. It was to get my lungs into better shape before surgery and then make them stronger as I recovered. The amount of lying down that I would be doing post-surgery would not be good for my lungs. The spirometer consists of a tube that you blow into, trying to keep a little ball inside suspended in the right position. As I like a challenge, I was rather pleased with it and practised a lot, trying each time to achieve a new personal best.

Surgery was booked for 12 days after my anaesthetist appointment. There is so much to do before an operation, which I hadn't realised. It was like preparing to go on the worst holiday ever, and you don't know what clothes to take or how long you'll be away for. As my car was usually kept on the street and I knew I wouldn't be able to drive for several weeks post-op, I left it on my sister's drive. That in itself was slightly painful. I love driving, love the independence it gives, and was nervous about when I would be able to drive again.

My elder son made arrangements for a holiday from work and for somewhere to stay in Derby. Very fortuitously, he was able to stay with my nephew, who lives a few miles out of Derby.

So, eventually, bags were packed and I was nearly ready. Both sons, Will and Dan, arrived the weekend before for a last hurrah. A friend drove a round trip of over 200 miles to pop in and bring me gifts. One was a crocheted pink penis, just to cheer me up. My sons and I had a fabulous time doing some of the things we have loved over the years. We went to an interesting BBQ–tapas style place for lunch, we watched *Top Gun* and *Hot Fuzz*, went for walks and played a couple of sessions of laser tag. I was shot many times. It was such a lot of fun and I was so happy to be with them.

We set off early to be at the hospital for 7 a.m. on the Sunday morning. It's so nerve-wracking hoping you've got everything right, not helped by the doors being locked at the clinic I had been asked to report to. At last, someone arrived and the processing started. Eventually, too, I was given a cubicle and the blood transfusions began. I can't remember how many litres I was given but it went on all day and into the night. Where does it go? Surely there must be a limit as to how much your veins can take before they start bulging out? Apparently not. I had been proud of myself as a good citizen for having been a blood donor in the past. The thirty litres I had donated had seemed a magnificent contribution. Now it seemed pretty paltry, when I realised how much can be used by one patient in one session.

Saying goodbye to my sons the night before the op felt pretty emotional. Would I see them again? What would I be like the next time I saw them? They had already been warned about how I would look when I was in ITU with wires and machines attached. The final goodbyes were gut-wrenching. And then I was on my own, just me and my bag of blood to contemplate the future.

The day of the surgery started early, with visits from surgeons and anaesthetists from 7 a.m. onwards. So far, so good. They just had to check the ITU situation to make sure there would be a bed available for when surgery was complete. I was on tenterhooks, and as time went on I became convinced it would not happen. But surely, they wouldn't send me home after all that blood and resources on their part? Finally, about 11 a.m., it was all go and I was whisked away. Here we go.

Obviously, I can't give you a first-hand commentary about the op. It was all in the hands, literally, of the surgical team. Elder son Will was down as point of contact and had organised a WhatsApp group for passing on information. This was a terrible waiting game for everyone else. The thread I subsequently saw showed a series of messages saying that there was no news yet and I was still in surgery. At last, the message came at 22:19 that the bulk of the surgery was done and they were just closing me up. The surgeon reported that 'all visible cancer was removed. The disease in the pelvis was very, very extensive and they had fitted a stoma'. As well as all the gynae bits, they had removed my gall bladder, the omentum and a lot of my lymph nodes.

I arrived in ITU just before midnight. The surgical team must have been exhausted. I was kept asleep until the following afternoon and then was given all of the information about the outcome. In fact, I think I was told several times and I knew I was happy about it, but still kept forgetting the details.

My main concern at this point was that my eyes didn't seem to be working properly. I kept saying that my eyes were like an old television where the picture kept slipping. I repeated it to anyone who would listen, and anyone who didn't, because I was worried my sight would be like that forever and no one seemed to be taking this seriously. I realise now that no one in the ward team was old enough to have seen a TV where you had to manipulate the vertical and horizontal hold knobs to keep the picture steady. I think they also probably knew that it would clear up once I was off the opiates. Indeed, after a few days my vision held steady and I no longer needed to think about adjusting the knobs.

Those first few days after the operation remain a blur to me, but I was moved to the high dependency step-down ward after about 36 hours. Gradually, tubes started to be removed. Thankfully, the one into my nose came out fairly early on. The teams are exceptionally skilled and although I was uncomfortable and possibly in some pain, it was taken very seriously and well controlled. I can't remember much about the pain now. They say when you have a baby that you forget the pain afterwards. I have never forgotten the pain of childbirth, but I have forgotten the surgical pain. I can't pretend it was lovely, though. I was trying to eat but couldn't because I was so nauseous. I was trying to sleep but couldn't, at least not at the right time. I vomited in the night, which strained my wound and made it bleed. Even so, the physios kept returning to get me out of bed and to encourage walking, or even just being upright. At this point, I was shocked by how weak and infirm I had become. I remember sitting on the edge of the bed, the chair just beside me, and having no idea how I was going to make it from one to the other. My body was no longer mine to command.

Over the next few days, more tubes were removed and the physios kept returning. I was so disappointed whenever I couldn't do what they asked because of my balance or my strength. They always said I was doing really well. I didn't believe them.

A fearful time was the threat to remove the catheter. Clearly, it had to come out at some point, and sooner was better than later, but how was I going to get to the bathroom? I was terrified that I would wet myself.

However, the nurse did remove it, and with support I made it to the toilet. More tubes were removed, including the one that would administer IV pain relief. After the catheter removal, this was my next big fear. It meant I would have oral pain relief instead. More on this issue later, but my fear of tablet-taking meant that I tended not to ask for pain relief unless desperate.

Eventually, ten nights after surgery, having passed my stoma test, ward-walking and stair-climbing tests, they said I was ready for discharge. It took a while to pack my bags given that I still felt very weak and was not allowed to lift anything. I should have remembered previous experiences with my mum's discharges from hospital that you can't actually leave until pharmacy have prepared your 'TTOs', the medication to take home. I'm not sure what the problem is, but it seems to be a perpetual issue that patients wait hours to be discharged because their medication hasn't arrived on the ward. I've no idea whether it's a communication issue between ward and pharmacy, a shortage of pharmacists or something else, but it is very frustrating. I was ready for discharge at 2 p.m. I had a two-hour journey home. My brother and sister-in-law were at my bedside waiting, ready to drive me back. No meds arrived. My rehab was improved during this time because I kept pacing the ward in frustration. I asked the nurses every hour if there was any sign of my meds. There wasn't. I had seen on the internet that the pharmacy closed at 7 p.m., so I presumed they would arrive before that. However, 7 p.m. came and went. I was tired and upset. At 7:30 p.m. I returned to the nurses' station and said I was going home without my meds and no, I couldn't pop back in the morning. Miraculously, two minutes later a bag of medication with my name on it turned up. I was free. The whole team had been amazing, but I was desperate to be home.

THE COLOSTOMY, ANOTHER SHITTY THING

What a surprise this one was. Before the surgery, I didn't really know what a stoma was. When I met the surgeon and he talked me through the long list of risks and effects of the surgery, this came out of the blue. He said a colostomy was likely. 'Likely?' I asked, hoping he would say that it was maybe a slight possibility. 'Likely,' he repeated. Shit, that sounded like he was saying it was more likely than not. It was the only thing he said that made me cry. He passed me the tissues. Then I went off with the very lovely nurse who let me cry a bit more. I imagined a long bottle strapped to my leg filled with piss and shit. The lovely nurse said I would meet the stoma nurse who would tell me all about it. Indeed I did on my next pre-op visit. The stoma nurse could not have been kinder or more clear about it all. She knew the image I had in my head. She showed me a stoma bag and a model of what the stoma itself would look like. She even gave me a plastic one to take home with me as a gift. I didn't display it on the mantelpiece.

'It's just a little bag on your tummy,' she reassured me. *No*, I thought. *It's a bag of shit on your tummy; it's not a place for keeping your Maltesers.*

She drew a circle on each side of my abdomen, ready for the surgeons, one for if I was to have a colostomy and one for if I had an ileostomy. I didn't want to think about it, although I made sure anyone involved in the surgery knew I wanted them to avoid it if possible. As with everything else though, it was the usual refrain of, 'Well, better that than dead.' I wonder what it would take for me to think that actually it might be better to be dead. I guess at some point I will find life and the treatment too unbearable to continue.

When I woke up after the surgery, having clocked that I was still alive, I was told that I'd had a colostomy. Looking back, my memory is that I took this rather prosaically. However, Will, who was by my bedside, said that every time I woke I would ask how the operation went and would be really happy. I would then ask if I had a stoma, and when he said yes, I would be really upset. Eventually, after asking these questions about five times, on my next awakening he told me that they had managed to save my legs. Apparently I reacted as though this was the funniest thing anyone had ever said. Clearly my brain was not functioning well after all the anaesthetic and the morphine.

The following day, the stoma nurse visited. The two stoma nurses were phenomenal, visiting daily, taking me through everything I needed to do to manage the stoma and repeating it until I cottoned on. It was no trouble at all for several days as nothing happened—very common, I was told. Then my stomach started to get quite uncomfortable and I was prescribed some medication to loosen my stools. Still nothing. The male stoma nurse thought an enema might help. However, unlike a normal enema, which goes up your bum and stays there, due to peristalsis (a word I hadn't heard since O Level Biology), the enema might suddenly pop out, so he had to put the tablet in my stoma and then hold it in with his finger while we chatted. So there I was, lying on my hospital bed, curtains around us, my gown up round my waist and the stoma nurse with his finger in what was now, for all intents and purposes, my front bum. That's when the student nurse walked in. I know it's difficult with curtains instead of doors, but I'm not sure just saying 'knock, knock' solves the privacy problem.

Two days later, nine days after the surgery, the stoma was definitely working. That was humiliating and outdid my worst fears. Fortunately I got to the bathroom, but it was everywhere. It looked as though shit had literally hit the fan. I didn't know where to start on cleaning up myself, my clothes and the bathroom. Amazing nurses came to the rescue again. They got just minorly irritated with me trying to help as I was getting in the way and probably spreading more around. They cleaned me up and said to leave the bathroom to them. Wonderful women, not a job I could do.

Since then, I have managed the colostomy OK in the main, and the service I received from the hospital stoma nurses, local stoma nurses and the stoma suppliers has been second to none. It still causes surprises though. Every so often, I still have to go to the loo to pass some sort of gunge which doesn't get as far as the stoma. Normal, I'm told. Between you and me, I quite like it. I miss having a proper poo. Getting that feeling, going to the loo and feeling better and emptier afterwards. You don't know what you've got till it's gone, apparently. I never thought a normal working bowel would be one of those things.

I've only had a few nasty events with it since, and initially I blamed either the Pfizer Covid jab or possibly pub cola for giving me diarrhoea. On one occasion, I thought my stoma sounded and felt a bit active, and I would normally go to the loo to check, but unfortunately, I was at a comedy club in the back room of a pub. If you've been to one of these things, you know you don't draw attention to yourself. You certainly don't stand up and leave the room without the risk of being questioned by the on-stage comedian. What would I say? 'Sorry, just got to change my colostomy bag.' It would have to be a very quick-witted comedian who had a funny retort for that one.

I whispered to my partner, asking if he could smell anything. 'Room just smells a bit musty,' he replied. I thought I could smell something. Perhaps it was a nearby smoker. I tried bending down to get closer, like you do when you suspect your baby has a full nappy. I couldn't be sure. I put my hand just under my top. It was damp. I rushed from the room. I was not questioned.

Fortunately there were lovely toilets, each with a washbasin. I stripped off and managed to clean up. Thank goodness for the spare knickers in my handbag. That was the end of the comedy night though. Nothing seemed that funny after that.

I have had a few 'poonamis' since then and have tried to identify what causes them. I have carried out experiments with avocado, mushrooms and, my latest theory, artificial sweeteners. At this point though, I can only conclude that Sid Stoma has a life of his own and I can't totally predict what he might do.

There are a few challenges with a colostomy. One nuisance is all the stuff you have to carry round with you. I keep buying new rucksacks in the hope that one of them will be ideal for storing the bags, wet wipes, dry wipes, adhesive remover, disposal bags, spare underwear, spare trousers. I gather from the colostomy Facebook group that airlines allow you extra on-board luggage allowance. Mind you, having explored the cost of travel insurance now, my foreign holidays may be at an end. I could afford either the insurance or the holiday but not both.

Yet another problem is 'pancaking'. My surgery was a couple of weeks before Pancake Day and I was confused by the colostomy Facebook group. Lots of laughing emojis and comments about being the kings and queens of pancakes. What? Then it dawned on me what they were talking about. Much of the time, the poo does not slide neatly down into your colostomy bag. It squashes itself around the entrance like a cowpat, getting bigger until there is a danger it will squash out of the sides. There are several solutions to this, none of which have been completely successful for me. You can put a sticker over the air vent. I had wondered what the little blue stickers were for in each box of bags and thought it was for a do-it-yourself star chart. Of course, you have to know where the air vent is on the bag, and I wasted several stickers by putting them in entirely the wrong place. The obvious drawback to covering the vent is that the bag fills up with air, expanding until you look like an over-excited male gorilla. There would certainly be no danger of drowning if you fell into a river. Other solutions are baby oil in the bag to help the poo slip down, or a ball of tissue to keep the bag slightly open. None of them have been all that helpful for me, but I guess they are for some people.

Another challenge is having a shower. Colostomy bags are waterproof so you can technically have a shower whilst wearing one. I tried that and really did not like having a wet thing flapping around the top of my thighs. I don't know how men put up with it. So, I've gone for the totally exposed stoma approach. But you do have to keep an eye on it. In my experience, the stoma, whom I have variously called Cilla, Sid, Stan and Colin, depending on our relationship, waits till you have shampoo on your head and soap in your eyes. Then it makes its move. Silent but deadly. You try and squint downwards through soap-agitated eyes and see it's on its way. You try and catch it. You try and get out of the shower without losing anything, dripping, but not able to put a towel round you. Showering becomes an extreme sport, adrenaline-fuelled, requiring speed, concentration, athleticism. Failure is literally shit.

Despite my initial fears, however, I have mainly come to terms with the stoma. I don't love it, but we do co-exist. I've been helped by all of those other 'ostomates' recently who have done amazing things and been proud to show their stoma bags. I haven't swum the English Channel, but I have started going to aqua-aerobics. The first few times I kept an eye on the water around me. Was there a big turd floating down towards the deep end, or a brown slick surrounding me? Would the pool have to be cleared and emptied? There was none of these things. I haven't shown off my stoma bag. In fact, I have worn a bathing costume, swim shorts and a support belt. However, aqua-aerobics is my equivalent of swimming the Channel.

IDENTITY

I guess one of the most surprising things about this 'adventure'—yes, I'll call it 'adventure' for a while, the ride of a lifetime, or the ride to end a lifetime. As I was saying, the most surprising thing—well, it's a surprise to me—is that I'm not who I thought I was. Or I have become someone who I can't relate to, and that makes me angry. We'll come on to anger in more detail a bit later, but boy, have I been angry.

Identity is a big deal these days. I've never really been into identity politics, or maybe I have but it wasn't called that. I've always been a feminist, a quite timid one I have to say. In more recent years I've also realised how much being from a working-class background has shaped me. Lack of self-belief, never feeling as good as the wealthy girls, never thinking my opinion counted for anything. But, I digress. Over the years I have got a bit more confident. I can give presentations to large groups of people. I could make significant decisions at work and at home, although always plagued by imposter syndrome. The one thing I have always believed about myself is that I am independent and can make my own choices. I have also realised in more recent years that this is not because I am a strong fearless woman, quite the opposite. I have been very easily influenced in the past, particularly by some men, giving up the good, decent ones and prone to bend towards the risky ones, paying undue attention to their opinions. I wonder if it's partly to do with going to an all-girls high school. While it may have been great for me academically, it probably hampered me socially. I never really got used to boys as ordinary creatures. For that reason, it's best for me to live alone so I don't just succumb to doing whatever someone else thinks I should do or, even worse, what I think they think I should do. I have a very supportive partner now, and although we are committed to one another we don't live together. I can't give up that hard-fought independence.

Long story short, then, I've been independent so I could do what I wanted. So, imagine what a shock it has been that I have needed to depend on people. This is not me.

It's taken a while to sink in, to realise that I am no longer a healthy, independent woman. Several months into all this, I was asked by a medical professional if I had any long-term conditions or was on any medication. 'No,' I said, then of course realised that I did. 'Well, yes, no, apart from the chemotherapy and the injections and the steroids and anti-coagulants and blood pressure medication. But I'm fine.'

Don't get me wrong—I was never really, really fit, been verging on overweight for a while, but I could run and walk and do whatever I wanted. I needed no help. Now I did. Just prior to my initial treatment, I could barely walk at all, having to rest every few yards. After my surgery, I found taking any steps difficult and frightening. Where had 'me' gone? I didn't recognise this person.

The lack of independence hit me hard. I felt ashamed. I wanted everyone to go away so that I could look after myself, even though I couldn't. At the beginning of this, when my sons and one of my nieces wanted to call up services and say I needed urgent treatment, I was appalled. No, I don't need people to speak for me. I would wait my turn, not be a nuisance, and sort things out myself. Eventually, I realised I didn't have the energy or the personal strength to do this and agreed for others to help. Lucky I did, as without their advocacy I might not be here to tell this tale.

It's a strange thing, this identity stuff, because in some ways you don't know what your identity is until it's threatened or aspects of it are taken away from you. I remember when I retired from work, it took a while to accept the label of 'retired'. I had been so much my job, which had carried with it a certain interest or respect from other people. When I retired, I was now just another older person—so, dull. But then I started doing more interesting stuff again—another degree, more exercise, personal challenges—so I felt OK about myself. Then this thing hit and I could see no hope of being that person again. Now I was just a person with cancer, end of. When you've got cancer, it is all-consuming. The majority of my brain is now taken up with cancer; it is the prism through which I see everything. I don't want it to be like this, but I'm having trouble changing it.

At this point, over a year in, most of the things I do each day don't involve my illness but it's rarely out of my head. When people ask how I am, I want to reply that I've got cancer. But I don't need to. Surprisingly, for a very private person, it's hard not to tell people in the street that I've got cancer. The strange thing is that, at the moment, I'm not even sure how much cancer I have. The surgery removed 'all visible cancer' and the blood tests are within normal range. But I'm still having treatment and I still feel debilitated compared with how I used to be. So, the identity I had just got used to, of being 'woman with cancer', may not be true either. I'm having to get used to a new, somewhat confusing, me.

The psychological dependency was something else. I have always sorted things out on my own. I think I am probably quite a secretive person, afraid of being judged or influenced. This changed a lot after my second divorce—yes, second—still embarrassed by my marriage failures. I needed people at that time as the whole debacle could no longer be kept under wraps. With cancer, too, there is little chance of hiding it. In a way, this is good. If I could have hidden it then, I would have done. I would then not have received the overwhelming support that has come my way and helped so much. I suppose this is the one thing that I have learned, that I need to talk to people who care about me. I don't really want to be helped, and initially felt that saying that I was OK would mean people would leave me alone. Well, that didn't work. It's been made clear to me that when my nearest and dearest ask me how I am, they really want to know. I try now to be clear about how I am feeling, and if they ask, then I tell them if I have been feeling a bit queasy or tired or fed up. Putting on a brave face is a really unhelpful thing to do.

THOSE DAMNED FEELINGS: ANGER, FEAR, ANXIETY AND HOPE

I guess I should be writing about all of the range of emotions that I've passed through in the last few months, the sadness and the fear, but I'll start with anger because, certainly for the first few months, anger was the most overwhelming and all-encompassing emotion. When I first had the diagnosis, I was furious, filled with rage. I wanted to just shout 'fuck', and did so quite a lot. My fury spilled out in all sorts of places. With cancer, there is nothing to direct it at. You can't be angry at cancer; it's just a thing that grows inside you. I couldn't blame anyone else for it. I wasn't sure if I could blame myself for it, although obviously I did try my best and thought around that one a bit. So, the main places my anger was directed were Coventry social services and Liz Truss.

My cousin, who has learning disabilities, for whom I was next of kin, had been in hospital and was discharged to a nursing home without our knowledge, and not back to the home he had been living in for many years. Phone calls and emails contained the full force of my anger, justified, but I probably did them with more relish than was required.

My second target, Liz Truss, had just become leader of the Tory party. Every time she appeared on TV, I was beside myself with fury. If I'd had the strength to march in demonstrations, I would have done.

A friend asked if I could think of lovely things instead to help me feel better. The answer was no. The anger was just bubbling and bubbling, and in the main these were two worthy recipients. Indeed, my wise sister encouraged it. In the early days, when mornings were worse for feeling bad and the deadly thoughts were gnawing around my head, she would say brightly, 'Shall we watch the news?' It worked. I could focus my anger outside myself rather than letting it eat up my insides along with the cancer.

Fear was and is another of my top emotions. There is the specific fear of a procedure, for example. In the early days, there were the tests to clarify the diagnosis, the colonoscopy, the range of scans, the biopsy, as well as the treatments, the pleural tap, the pleural drain. Then there is the anxiety as you wait to be told the results of all of these. As well as the specific fears, there is also a general anxiety that never really goes away, it just ebbs and flows. I used to have such confidence in my body. If I had a sniffle, I could be pretty confident it would be gone the next day. It made me feel invincible. How foolish I feel now, when for so long this thing must have been growing inside me. Once that confidence had gone, I was left with the feeling that anything could go wrong at any time. There were always additional organs or complications that had never crossed my mind before that were involved or might be affected. I could not believe how many organs were removed in my surgery. I thought they were just taking out a lump in my abdomen. In fact, there were so many that I still can't recall everything that was actually removed. So to my mind now, anything could happen at any time. I'm only one blood test away from bad news.

The general anxiety is there all the time. When I wake in the morning it's my first thought. It wasn't a nightmare, this is reality. Then the anger comes back. Fuck, fuck, fuck, fucking cancer. It feels like a surprise every day. Of course, whilst you're lying in bed, there is so much opportunity to travel down rabbit holes. Ruminating has always been a problem for me, and now it's my main hobby. What if, what if, what if... Of course, it doesn't take much to bring out the whole playlist. Palpitations, eh? Well, you're probably going to have a stroke. Urgency for the toilet, eh? Probably kidney damage. You've lost a bit of weight? Well, the cancer has come back. You've put on a bit of weight? Well, that's not going to help stave off the cancer, is it?

I generally decide I have only a few days left to live and must make sure I tidy up. For some reason, leaving things in order is my main preoccupation. I asked my CNS one of my 'what if' questions one day. She said simply, 'Well, if that happens we'll deal with it.' I have to try and remember this when I'm feeling panicky. They are experts and they will deal with it.

One of my biggest discoveries of the last year, and one that other people probably already knew, is the importance of hope. People have said to me in the past that I am a very positive person. I'm not sure I am. I like to think of myself as a realist rather than an optimist. I'm not a glass half full or half empty person, I'm a 'that line there is how full the glass is' person. But I realise now that I have always been hopeful. If things are bad then there must be a way of sorting them out, even if it takes a while. I guess that's because I am lucky to have had loving, encouraging parents, a good education and to have been born at a time when we thought things would always get better. I worry now about the lack of hope around, particularly for young people. If your only hope to better yourself is to be a drugs runner or to set off in a small boat to the other side of the world then perhaps many of us would do that, just to maintain a bit of hope.

For me, hope suddenly disappeared from my life. I was going to die, and quite soon. All the statistics I had read said that. The A&E doctor had said that. I was a lost cause. During the summer before my diagnosis was finalised and any treatment had started, I asked my niece, who had been a Macmillan nurse in the past, what would happen if the oncologist said there was nothing they could do. 'Oh, they won't say that,' she replied. I could hardly believe it, but it was just a glimmer that all was not lost.

For most of those summer months, I tried to hang on to that tiny spark, but it was tough. It wasn't just that I had no hope, but also that I dared not believe I might have hope. I couldn't bear the thought that if I felt too hopeful it was a fool's errand, bound to end in crushing disappointment. I could not think about the next Christmas; I could not think about planning anything more than a few days away because I was convinced I would not be around. I can tell you, it is hard to live without hope.

Over the last few months, I have started to feel hopeful again. The evidence before me suggests I am doing OK and that I have longer to live. I still do not know how long, but the fact that I've lasted a year longer than I thought has given me great hope and a feeling that I've cheated the cancer, even if only for a short time. There is a bit of adrenaline that goes with that. It's as if I've ridden at speed round a corner on my motorbike and not fallen off. Well, I never managed that, but so far, so good on the cancer.

Thinking about these emotions more recently, it struck me that I have been going through the stages of grief. There are many models of grief, but I had certainly been through shock, anger, numbness, depression, sometimes acceptance, and then back through them all again. It was as though I had already died and I was grieving myself, even to the point of planning my funeral. Realising this turned out to be helpful. I suddenly grasped that, surprise, surprise, I am not yet dead, so grieving myself was unnecessary and pointless. Yes, I know I'm also grieving the years I won't have and that's reasonable, but to grieve my own death was a step too far.

It is so easy to sink into the feelings: the panic, the fear of the future. When I recognise this happening now, I try and ground myself, to look around, to see, to smell, to listen to what is around me. I repeat to myself, 'I am here. I am alive.' It's a surprisingly good sensation, to remember that.

REHAB, RECOVERY, OR JUST HOW TO SPEND YOUR LIMITED TIME

When you think about how much time you've got left at any stage in your life, you might have a wish list. Perhaps a bucket list of things you want to do, experiences you want to have, maybe things you want to achieve. Anyway, it all seems so far away, no need to rush.

Then it happens. There is no more time. Or perhaps a very short amount of time. Or you often don't know how much time. So what do you do? Well, here's the thing. I haven't rushed around booking adventures, even when I've felt relatively well. I haven't written the novel. Because not much matters. I feel that perhaps I ought to make TikTok videos or do some sort of physical feat so I can inspire people and they can say how brave I was and set up a fund in my memory. Hats off to those who do that, you have my full admiration, but drawing attention to myself has never really been me. To be fair, I do like attention, but I could never ask for it. I never used to speak in lessons or even give my opinion on anything, but I would have so loved to be chosen. I might have died of embarrassment, but that was what I secretly hoped for: to be noticed. But I never have been.

I have never really made an impact in a crowd. That's why I used to love acting. I could be centre stage without having to worry about saying the wrong thing, because they weren't my words. You wouldn't believe how many funny retorts I could have made in meetings or in conversations if only I'd had the courage. I'm not a brave person, but both of my sons are. I don't know how they do it; they are magnificent. Occasionally, after a glass of wine I become a bit more extroverted and think at the time that I have been brilliantly funny. Then later that night I wake up in a cold sweat. Who have I upset? Did I talk to everyone I should have? Did everyone there think I was stupid? Then I will get flashbacks over the next few days, maybe weeks or months, of something I'd said, or not said.

So, no big demonstrations of bravery or inspiring challenges or trips for me.

It's also very exhausting having cancer. Even when I've felt OK, once I have got up off the sofa or done a little job then I am knackered again. It's not even a normal tiredness; it's a feeling of not really being bothered or capable of doing much more. It seems such a waste.

So what do I do? Sadly, I have spent quite a bit of my limited time watching TV. I love all of those police investigation programmes. Something about people getting their comeuppance. I should have been a police officer. I tried, but it was in the days when there was a height restriction and policewomen had to be at least five foot four inches and I was only 5 foot three. I'm even shorter now, so presumably would have been dismissed at some point. Nah, they don't really dismiss anyone, do they? I would have been a terrible police officer anyway. Too scared, too compliant and might have got sucked into a corrupt culture. So, I've been satisfied watching other people cleverly catching out scammers and murderers.

As well as TV watching, I have done lots of puzzles: Waffle, Wordle, Quordle, Octordle, how to waste your lifele. So, that's not really a good thing. Surely I should be doing marvellous things, not sitting on the sofa.

So, how can I get back to the me I was, or the new me as I want to be? One thing that helped with the physical dependence and rehab was having people who celebrated my small achievements, who reminded me of how far I'd come. 'Mum, I know you've only walked to the end of the road, but two weeks ago you were in intensive care.' Oh yes, I'd forgotten that. And, of course, the people who walked with me, literally and figuratively.

The second thing that helped was having small goals. In the hospital, after surgery, each day the doctors would say which tube was going to be removed next. I had a clear but scary plan of what needed to happen before I could be discharged. I needed to be able to walk down the corridor, go up and down stairs, manage my stoma. At last, things were in my control if I put some effort in. I did, and was released.

Since coming out of hospital post-surgery, I have tried to keep up the small steps. I was devastated and frightened on being told that having a colostomy meant I was a high risk for a hernia. It felt such a kick in the teeth. How on earth was I meant to get stronger when exercise would put a strain on my abdomen? I spent weeks imagining I had a hernia or was about to get a hernia. The stoma nurse organised for me to be fitted for a support belt. I guessed that was a good thing. I booked in to see a physio, who gave me exercises to very slowly build up my core and general strength without putting too much strain around the stoma. So far, so good. No hernia and I'm feeling stronger. It's good having something that is in my control, something I can do.

There is so much done to you when you have cancer, so much that you don't comprehend. I have always thought I could understand what medical sites were saying, but I've realised that my understanding of anatomy, drugs and treatment options is miniscule. More than that, though, is that I am sometimes too scared to do any research about these things because the statistics are often frightening and demoralising. It feels better for me to stick my head in the sand and do what I can control, so a few more squats and dead lifts.

One of the ways I have spent my time is walking. Way before all this shit, I signed up for a Conqueror Challenge and the one I chose was a virtual Lands End to John O'Groats walk. It was called LEJOG. For the first six months, I thought it was French and would pronounce it with a French accent, then someone pointed out what the letters stood for. LEJOG is an app on your phone with an avatar that moves as you record your daily steps, or they are recorded automatically via an app like Google Fit. I had started off well, although Cornwall is clearly a lot bigger than I had thought. Then I became ill. When I had so much fluid in my pleural cavity that I needed a rest halfway up my stairs, I never thought I would walk more than a few steps again. I presumed I would be stuck forever in a virtual Dorset. Walking means a lot to me, though. It means freedom, independence, getting somewhere without being reliant on anyone or anything. It also means I can be in nature. My local park, Abington, just at the end of the road, is wonderful. We are so lucky that places like this were created or donated in the last couple of centuries. I know their origins in the Industrial Revolution shouldn't make me too grateful, but I'm so happy that park is there. When breathing, walking and the need for the loo made it almost impossible to get there, I was desperate. Eventually, I managed to get to the end of the road, and then to the outskirts of the park, then to the first bench, etc. Getting out to proper countryside is even better. Passing the sign that says 'Brecon Beacons' makes me breathe more easily. It's one of my favourite places and I want to go again and see the sign that says 'Bannau Brecheiniog'.

To get back to LEJOG—what a great motivator that turned out to be. I had started off in Cornwall in the rudest of health, or so I thought. A few months in and I could barely walk. Suddenly, my fluid-filled pleural cavities and the mass pressing on my bowel meant that I struggled to breathe and needed the loo at frequent and unpredictable intervals. I was sad that I would never finish. However, as I improved with treatment and got stronger, I managed more walking. My little avatar on the app sometimes only moved a few steps each day but she gave me added motivation to add a few more steps. Eventually, about six months after I had originally planned, I completed the last three kilometres walking round a local reservoir and finished LEJOG. I had arrived at the virtual John O'Groats. It felt very much as though I really had walked from one end of Great Britain to the other. Even though I had walked it all in tiny steps, I was delighted with myself.

So, the main thing I have found helpful is to move my body, even though it's usually the last thing I want to do, mainly because of the tiredness and generally feeling lethargic the whole time. I have had a varied history with exercise. I have always liked doing exercise but never liked starting it. Once it was underway then I loved it and felt great afterwards. My solution has been to tell myself that all I have to do is to stand on the doorstep with my exercise kit on. That's the hard bit done. I have joined a number of gyms over the years and rarely got beyond the induction. I don't think I've ever been to one more than five times. Then I found outdoor exercise. I joined a military fit style exercise group. That sounds a bit more taxing and impressive than it really is. It is very much moulded to the abilities of the members, so the really fit people do lots more running and more repetitions of the exercises.

At times in the last year, I could barely move at all. This was from breathlessness, exhaustion or the fear of a hernia. The physio has been a bit of a godsend, giving me the confidence to get back to exercise without doing further harm, trying to improve my lung capacity and building up my strength. Gradually, I am starting to feel less like an old woman.

This has enabled me to return to my outdoor fitness. Where the exercises given in the session might put too much strain on me, I have done my own exercises. It doesn't really matter. What is important is that I have been outside, in the fresh air, in a beautiful park and moved my body. Most importantly, I have been with my friends. Some of them I have known for a long time and they have been in touch throughout my illness, supporting me and encouraging me.

Another way of spending my time, which has been enormously helpful, has been walking football. I haven't fully returned to it yet, just been to a couple of short training sessions, but it's there in my goals, literally.

I have also read a few books. This has been a challenge in itself. I used to love reading and it took a lot to drag me out of a book once I was into it. Now, my concentration is a bit non-existent. Fortunately, I already belonged to a book club, and while I couldn't read at all at some points in the last year, once I started going back to the book club then the extra motivation of wanting to contribute made me set aside time to read. Of course, books take you to a different time, a different place, get you into the soul of a different person. What a relief. At the worst times, I could listen to some of the books and other stories on Audible. Wonderfully distracting.

NOT JUST ABOUT ME

So far this has been all about me. But cancer affects everyone who knows you, who loves you. What I have found is that it is so difficult to know what to do about other people or even to think about other people while all this is happening. Sometimes my head is so full of the fact I have cancer that there seems no room for anyone or anything else. Initially, before my diagnosis, I wasn't going to tell anyone else that I thought there was something wrong. I didn't want anyone else giving me their opinion or telling me what I ought to do. And, of course, it couldn't be anything that bad...

Telling my sons was my biggest concern. They are grown men, but I am still their mum and my role is to be there for them, celebrating their successes, sharing their worries, if they want me to. But here I was, about to make their lives so much worse, the very opposite of what I wanted. I wasn't going to tell them until I was absolutely sure, because why would I worry them unnecessarily? This was when my niece Sally stepped in. My sister had told her about the tests as she had been a nurse. Sally's opinion was very clear, that I needed to tell my sons what was happening, sooner rather than later, pointing out that they would be really upset if I kept it from them and they had been unable to support me. She was right. And in a way it was easier to tell them when there was nothing definite, when it was just having a few tests, even though we all knew deep down that the outcome wasn't going to be a quick fix.

Neither of my sons lives near me or near each other, each living in cities at opposite ends of the country. I couldn't pop in to see them and explain over a cup of tea, so it meant messaging and asking if they had time to talk. My elder son, Will, said that this rang alarm bells. He remembers being stood in a friend's child's paddling pool at the time. He told me later that he found the conversation quite disorientating as I played it down massively, but it was clear I thought something was wrong. This left him with a feeling that perhaps he couldn't be trusted and that I didn't believe him to be adult enough to deal with it. He asked me to record my next appointment, which was with the bowel consultant. He found the recording hard to listen to because he could tell how frightened I was. I, of course, had thought I was calm and composed. He contacted Sally at that point, who explained about ovarian cancer and the implications. He said it felt like being punched in the gut.

My younger son, Dan, also has a clear memory of my call. He was out for a walk. He said he could hear that I was battling to present a calm, composed front but that my voice cracked slightly. He described the feeling of the entire world shifting around him, that he had dropped five foot and landed in the same spot.

Looking back, it might have been better to tell them earlier, not just because they are adults but because I'm pretty sure they would have told me to get it investigated quicker, rather than delay. They would certainly not have allowed me to use the excuse of the GP surgery not having any appointments.

Thank goodness I took Sally's advice and told them earlier than I might, because they have been an immense support and the last year has brought us even closer. I think one of the things that has helped me is that, when I have not been in critical stages of my illness, they have still told me all about their lives, how work has been going, their friendships, the details of their days. Best of all, they still seem interested in my views, although I have always been very cautious about giving them my opinion ever since they became teenagers. I wonder if they continue to be protective of me and don't tell me things they think would worry me too much. They probably talk more to each other now, even though they live so far apart. And that's got to be a good thing, because, whatever my outcome, I'm not going to live forever and it's a nice thought, for me, that they will have each other as well as their myriad friends and family.

This has been an immensely tough time for them, though. I have asked them more recently what it has been like. Even though we are really close, there are so many things unsaid in relationships and so many assumptions made. I guess as well, we don't always know ourselves what is going on inside until we are able to articulate it. My sons have many similarities: they are funny, generous, loving and with strong values. They are also very different in the way they go about things. Will has to sort things out quickly, make things right, rally the troops. Dan is calm, measured, taking time to process the best course of action. Dan said that initially this brought a feeling of guilt as it was Will doing all the work and making things happen. Having spoken to me and his partner, he realised his role was important too: seeing me, talking to me, being with me in all senses.

Both felt that what was helpful was 'being in the room', that they knew what was going on, as much as any of us did. They also valued each other and being able to share; being aware that the other knew what it all felt like was 'a real comfort'. They also had other family and friends around them, who were exceptionally supportive.

Dan described it as a 'stark reminder of what's important'. This has made us all think about how far apart we are from one another geographically. They both have busy jobs and social lives, so time together is limited. If you're looking at a shortened lifespan then, as Will pointed out, 'This means that the times we have together in the future might be counted in dozens rather than hundreds.' They both felt some guilt, unnecessarily in my opinion, that we don't necessarily see each other a lot, although we have some weekends and the annual wonderful family holiday. They do, however, phone regularly and always have done, either every day or at least every couple of days. These aren't quick calls, they are long, meaningful conversations, so for me, not being with them in the flesh isn't a huge issue. I don't think we could be more close.

This thing has changed all of us. It gives a new perspective. None of us are special in the great scheme of things. There are no guarantees. We have become both more resilient and more vulnerable. What has helped is being able to show that vulnerability in front of one another, believing that sharing those feelings is OK. We can trust each other that, one way or another, we can deal with whatever emotion or challenge comes our way.

I have always known I am fortunate to be part of a large, supportive family. Having never expected to be ill, and being the youngest sibling, I had always thought it would be me in the future who would do the helping. Now, it was all of them helping me. This was a tough concept to come to terms with. I'm not sure how I would have managed without them. My sister Yvonne didn't even ask what I needed. There was no querying what hours she should come. She was just there, doing it all when I was at my physical and emotional weakest, after every chemo session and after my surgery. She cooked, cleaned, talked, listened. At weekends, my partner came to stay, providing support and a listening ear to my fears. I wonder how other people manage when they haven't got such reinforcements.

There are so many other people. There are the very close ones, family and friends; there are people who you see a lot but you're not on intimate terms with; there are people you used to be really close to but now have only occasional contact with, and then there are people you see but have no investment in, such as neighbours, the hairdresser, the woman at the corner shop. It's so difficult to know what to say to people, and I'm sure many don't know what to say to me. It's odd, this greeting which has become so common: 'Y'alright?' Clearly to me, I am not alright. Even when I'm at my very best I still have cancer or am receiving cancer treatment. But I can't say, 'No, actually, I've got cancer and might die.' So, while in the past I used to respond, 'Yes, fine thanks, how are you?' I now say, 'Not too bad, thanks.'

People also, of course, all respond very differently to the news. Some want to know all the details—or perhaps that's because many of my friends have a physical or mental health background. They are fascinated by the story. Others make it clear that they want to know nothing. And that's fine; I just have to be aware of the signals and not unload information on people for my own benefit. A few have tried to say something to cheer me up, like they knew someone with cancer and they were fine. That has made me want to shout that I have a really shit form of cancer and I probably won't be fine. I don't say that, of course, I just nod and say, 'Oh good.' Most people offer to help and really genuinely want to, specifying things they can do: pick up prescriptions, come to chemo with me, get shopping, etc. You feel that these people mean it. One of the strangest ones was a neighbour who expressed sympathy and said as usual, 'Well, let me know if there's anything you need.' He added, 'Just put a note through the door.' I wondered what I could ask for in a note. An ambulance, a pint of milk? But none of us know what is really going on in other people's lives, and to be fair, I'm not sure I've ever offered to help them with anything either.

I have several groups of friends, people I have met from various stages of my life, career and hobbies. There are the 'Leicester Girls', the 'Forget-me-nots', the 'Very Old Friends', the 'Book Club' friends, the 'Fit for Purpose' friends, the 'Creative Writers' friends and the 'Walking Footballers' as well as many individual friends from different walks of life. I have been overwhelmed by the support I have received from all of them. People seem to feel a need to send a gift. This is unnecessary, but I can understand why. I guess people just want to do something tangible and there is very little they can do. I received so many thoughtful presents: books, calming lotions, pocket hugs and many bouquets of flowers. One of my teenage great-nieces, Emily, made a little clay heart, painted it red and wrote a beautiful message. I took that heart with me to some of my procedures when I was most scared and felt it in my pocket. It brought me comfort.

The 'Forget me-nots' took a different approach. Well, they are psychologists. From them I have received a succession of gifts, all around the theme of 'fuck off to cancer' or penises. I am surprised they were able to source so many gifts with this motto. There must be a special site on the dark web. So, I have fuck off socks, fuck off candles, fuck off china hearts, colouring books of penises and a pink crocheted penis. They certainly achieved the outcome of making me laugh, and they know that's what I love most.

Many friends have kept in touch. One has messaged me every day since this started. It might just be to say

'Morning' or it might be a little longer, but it is such a gesture of friendship. The Walking Footballers have messaged regularly and also invited me to events that I could manage: a coffee, an afternoon tea, a ride in a classic car, a crown green bowling session. I am one very lucky woman.

INFORMATION, GOOGLE SEARCHES AND SOCIAL MEDIA

I have always loved information, statistics, research. The internet is a wonderful thing if you use reputable sources and follow people who know what they are talking about. In the past, if I had a problem, then I would do a bit of research and find a plan of action. So, of course, the first thing I did after the question of ovarian cancer was raised was google it and look at medical sites. The omentum had been mentioned by the CNS, so I searched for that, just to find out what it was. I searched for about two minutes. The information I was reading about survival rates was horrific. They were talking about months. I slammed the laptop shut, my heart pounding, feeling that I couldn't breathe. I was beside myself with fear. It was as though I had inadvertently stepped into a cage without noticing the lion in there and had only just managed to escape. I knew I couldn't do that again.

From being a woman who wanted to know everything, I was now a woman who wanted to know nothing. Better to bury my head in the sand. I could not think about the future because it looked really shit. I still don't look at survival rates, but I have moved from planning how to get through the next hour to planning the next month.

Obviously, there are some fantastically helpful internet sites. Target Ovarian Cancer is one I look at occasionally and appears sometimes on my Facebook feed. I joined it as it was recommended to me by an ex-colleague who had the same diagnosis as me a year earlier. She clearly found it very helpful. It's an excellent website, but to be honest, when it appears on my Facebook feed, I generally have a quick look and then snooze it for another 30 days. I have to remind myself that the people who pose questions on there are the ones who want some help, not the ones who are managing OK. I can't cope with seeing things that have happened to other people because I then believe they will happen to me, and it knocks me down for a long time while I panic about it. I don't want to see these things. I only want the good news. Now, if I need to know something, I go directly to the reputable sites like Target Ovarian Cancer, Macmillan Cancer Support or Ovacome Ovarian Cancer. Then I can funnel my search into a specific question and not be diverted into terror.

The things that work for me online are the scientific presentations delivered by doctors and researchers. I really enjoy these. I can sit back, take notes of statistics, the science and anatomy of ovarian cancer, and learn about current research. I am switched into thinking I am listening to an interesting work project and not something that is life and death for me. One of the Target Ovarian Cancer online talks I went to opened with a short talk from a woman who'd had the same diagnosis seven years earlier. It was wonderful to hear at a time when I thought I only had weeks. Another little chink of hope appeared on my horizon. I have also been to a couple of their online creative writing sessions. These are a joy and a relief, and amazingly, attendees rarely mention cancer. There are so many other things to think about, all of them positive.

Having said all that about not looking at much online, I must probably make an exception for the Facebook group 'Colostomy UK support group'. While I also don't look at this regularly, I have found there is lots of helpful, practical advice. Even better is that the contributors seem to have humour which is right up my street. They are a very funny bunch. It's instructive too to see the pictures of children and young people with stomas who are dealing with this really well. It certainly takes away any chance of a 'poor me' on my part.

So, we all have to find our own way with social media. I guess some people find it helpful to be part of a community of those living with the same disease. I'm not that person. I can't be upset for other people; my own issue is enough. I want only very specific advice from an expert and only when I ask for it. I don't want to be walloped unexpectedly by information that is going to push me over. To be honest, I'm just trying to keep upright. That's hard enough in itself.

Of course, there's not just online information; there are good old-fashioned books and leaflets. Macmillan do a phenomenal range of helpful guides which are available in oncology waiting rooms and from their service. They are clear and well written, and give ways forward for whatever problem you are experiencing at the time. These feel so much more manageable than an internet site which can punch you in the face without warning.

THE BRCA GENE,
SOMETHING ELSE I'D NEVER HEARD OF

'Do you want to be tested for the BRCA gene?' asked the consultant at my very first appointment with him. I thought he probably had some research project going on and wanted some subjects. I had no idea about the significance of genetics to my condition. I answered, 'Yes, that's fine.' I had to fill in a huge questionnaire. Well, the questionnaire wasn't that huge but my family is, so that's what took all the time and some detective work. My mother was one of seven and my father one of eleven, so tracking down dates and causes of death was something of a challenge.

I didn't give it much thought after that. However, the results came back to say that I have a mutation of the BRCA1 gene. This was a complete shock. I couldn't look back in my family history and see a clear line of cancer at a particularly young age. While there was cancer in the family, you would not necessarily notice that it was more frequent than in anyone else's family. My paternal grandmother died in her early sixties of breast cancer, and my mum had breast cancer, identified early by a mammogram, when she was 70. Only one aunt had died still in middle age, and given how many aunts I have, that did not make any of us consider genetics.

But there it was, yet another surprise in this whole business. BRCA is a short way of saying BReast CAncer gene. People who inherit harmful variants in BRCA1 and BRCA2 have increased risks of several cancers. The genetic link was not good news, in that it means I have a high risk of the cancer recurring and in other parts, such as the breast. As a result, I was sent for a mammogram. I was also booked in for a breast scan, which I had never had before. What an experience that one was. I had to strip off my top and then lie face down on the scanning table. It was a bit like how when you go for a back massage there's a hole for your face, but in this case each breast had to fit through an individual hole. I felt as though I was either caught up in some sex contraption or I was a pig in a farrowing crate. Not my best look either way. Of course, during the wait for the tests and the results I convinced myself that I had breast cancer as well. Happily, all is well so far in that department, but I am on the high-risk list and will have a mammogram every year.

Maybe surprisingly, finding out there was a genetic component to my cancer made me feel a bit better. Firstly, it meant that this was not my fault. I didn't need to look for bad lifestyle choices I had made. Secondly, I felt I was taking one for the team. A bit like the canary in the mine. While I was very concerned that this meant my family could also have the gene, at least they could get tested and be alert for symptoms of breast, ovarian and prostate cancer. Finally, there are specific treatments for those with the BRCA gene. Drugs called PARP inhibitors are a type of targeted therapy. Not that it's important, but this stands for poly-ADP ribose polymerase. These inhibit the ability of damaged ovarian cancer cells to repair themselves. I now take twice-daily oral PARP inhibitors as well as three-weekly 'infusions' of bevacizumab in the chemo suite. I can only remember the name bevacizumab by transposing it into the Everly Brothers song 'Be-Bop-A-Lula' she's my baby... I sometimes sing it in my head as it is being infused into my veins. Somehow it cheers me up, as again, the side-effects aren't lovely. It has added to my peripheral neuropathy, I am exhausted, I get nose bleeds and mouth ulcers. But, I'll say it again: I'm still here.

SO, WHAT'S BEEN THE WORST BIT?

You might find this hard to believe because it is so ridiculous. The most troubling thing for me has not been the chemotherapy or the surgery. It's swallowing tablets. There, told you it's ridiculous. Actually, it's not just tablets. I've also struggled with swallowing the range of other substances they give you, like the pre-scan fluid or the magnesium supplements.

I have taken tablets in the past, but just occasional antihistamines, which are tiny. I think I'd only taken one paracetamol in my life before this. This is because I have been extremely fortunate with my health, and also because I'd rather have the minor ailment or pain than swallow a tablet. Yes, I'll say it again, ridiculous.

This might sound like a small thing and I know it's very hard for other people to contemplate why it's such a big issue for me. I have been given much advice. Just throw it to the back of your mouth and swallow, or just have a big glass of water. Yeah, why didn't I think of that. Or even worse, 'Look at me, I can swallow all mine at once without any water.' Well, I can't. It's not an understatement to say that it has dominated some of my days. I have now improved a bit in this whole tablet debacle, but for much of the last year I would wake up and, after having remembered, *Shit, I have cancer*, my next thought would be, *I've got to take those fucking tablets*. I would try and take them early in the morning so I could forget about it for the rest of the day. You can imagine my disappointment when I found out that I had to take the PARP inhibitors at night too.

I have done a bit of research on the issue and felt vaguely better that I'm not alone. I was greatly reassured that medication swallowing problems are associated with smaller mouth cavity size and higher density of taste receptors on the tongue. I knew it was because I'm such a delicate princess. Anyway, that didn't solve the problem, and I recognised it was probably both a physical and psychological issue. It's not something that can be easily tackled because the gag reflex is so strong. I had to be near a sink when I took some of the medication as I was likely to throw it up. I would take the most challenging tablets first so that if I retched then I wasn't jeopardising all of them. Then I thought: of course, I know how to deal with this—I'll draw up my own desensitisation programme. Stage 1: start with teeny weeny jelly tots cut up into teeny weeny pieces. I couldn't swallow them.

More research by me and helpful friends and family suggested that, while the temptation is to tilt your head back to swallow, it's much better to lean forwards. The most helpful technique we discovered is the pop bottle method. Put the tablet in your mouth and then slug down some fizzy drink from a bottle and the vacuum you create in the bottle will whoosh down the tablet. Well, usually.

As I said, I've got much better at it, but I still dread it. I don't need the pop bottle so much now. I have orange juice or milk, which deaden the taste. I never let the tablet touch the top of my mouth or the back of my tongue, and I hold my breath so I can't smell the most stinky one. I try and distract myself by listening to the radio or doing a crossword, and then I do it. Yes, still ridiculous, but that's the price you pay for being a princess.

THE END

I don't know what my ending will be like. If I think about it then I guess it might be painful and I will look like a dying woman. I'm not sure why the thought of my appearance bothers me. It's never been my primary concern, but somehow, I don't want my poor family and friends to have to remember me looking that bad.

I don't very often think about the end stages of my life as it is too frightening. Sometimes, however, it slaps you in the face. I was in the emergency assessment bay a few weeks ago for a check-up, and during the afternoon, the man in the chair next to me was visited by his consultant. Nothing is private in hospitals when you are only inches apart, and I heard the doctor say to him that perhaps it was time to involve the palliative care team because his continual cough might be better treated by them. I did not need more than a glance to see the impact this had on my fellow patient. Devastating. I wondered when I would be told that. Months, years?

There has been quite a bit in the news recently about assisted dying. I feel I ought to have an opinion on this but I am in two minds. I have worked a lot with older people and could imagine scenarios where someone feels such a burden that it would be easy to persuade them into it. I also can't imagine that I would ever voluntarily say goodbye to my family and close friends. My FOMO, fear of missing out, would trouble me too much. However, my hatred of dependency tends to lean me in the other direction. What about if I am in so much pain, or can't communicate? My feelings, of course, may well change.

At the moment, my sons have power of attorney if I lose my faculties. I have jotted down a few notes about what I would not like, but this is fairly limited and mainly consists of 'don't give me milky tea or bananas' and 'don't bring in dogs to comfort me or that might finish me off'. End of life decisions are a lot to put on my sons, but I trust that they know me well enough to make the right ones.

I sometimes think about my funeral. But to be honest, it's not for me. I know some people plan their own funeral in detail, but I think it is for others to do that. I'd just like it to be a good one. Choosing the music, the poetry, the clothes, the type of coffin are all part of the grieving process for those left behind. A chance to reminisce. So, I've made few specifications. I think a bit of time to cry and then a lot of time to laugh should be factored in. I couldn't care less to be honest. So, over to you for the rest of it. Oh, but just one more specification. Back to where I started this on phrases that really irritate me. I don't want anyone to say that I have 'passed'. What a meaningless phrase that is. Passed what? Wind? Kidney stones? Passed where? I don't think I'm going to be floating in the sky, although if it helps people to imagine that, then that's fine with me. I hope that people will just be told I've died. Much more unambiguous.

Anyway, I am not yet at the point of planning my end of life care. I am still being actively treated. I know things can change very quickly, and it wasn't that long ago that I thought I was about to die. Somehow, by the cleverness of researchers, the knowledge and care of the medical and nursing teams, and definitely by the love and determination of my family and friends, I am still here. That is such a bonus. When I look back on the last months,

I am so grateful. OK, a lot of it has been quite shit, but a lot of it has also been wonderful. The time I have spent with family and friends has been really special because we know how special it is. I have already done a lot of the things I wanted to do in my life. The rest of my family are healthy. I have had time to realise all of this and I have had time to put some things in order. Most recently, I returned to walking football and scored two goals. Once you've done that, I think you can say life is complete.

I now understand the number I was told by the A&E doctor who called me a 'Poor Lady'. It was my CA125, a measure of a particular protein and good at identifying ovarian cancer. Normal levels are less than 35. Mine at that time was over ten thousand. My latest blood test gave my CA125 as seven.

I started off writing this by thinking about hope. I now do have hope. It's not the hope for a long life. I don't know how much longer my life will be. It's the hope and expectation that whatever happens, my family and friends will support me through it. I am so lucky to have had this extra time with them. I'm sure there are a few nasty corners still to get round, but I haven't reached the end of the road yet. And I am loving the ride along with my gang.

ALIVE

I am alive
to the roar of the waterfall, crashing over the rocks
I am alive
to the warmth of a hug
I am alive
to the sight of my boys' names lighting up my phone
I am alive
to the sight of the fungus sprouting from the decaying tree
I am alive
to the breath-taking glory of the starling murmuration
I am alive
to the rain lashing my face
I am alive
to the laughter forcing its way through my chest
I am alive
to the colours of the trees covering the mountains
I am alive
to the anticipation of Christmas fun
I am alive.

EXTRA TIME

Many of the players are lying flat on the pitch.

They have given their all

stung with disappointment that it was not enough

leaving their fans with anguished faces and nail-bitten fingers.

They roll down their socks, physios massage their thighs and shins

until they drag themselves upright once more

to form the circle, arms over one another's shoulders,

seeking the energy, the motivation for just one more push

praying to finish before penalties,

praying that if it's not,

that they will not be the one who fails.

I remain upright, still standing,

not quite given my all

but still fearful, still anxious and worn by the effort.

My supporters are tired, drained but delighted with my extra time.

My socks are rolled down and my sleeves are rolled up.

Medics work on me, infusing the energy, instilling the motivation to keep going.

I am still on the field, still thrilled to be playing.

The final score is irrelevant,

just continue to keep playing,

I'll take the Russian roulette of penalties if needed.

They think it's all over,

Oh no it isn't.

ACKNOWLEDGEMENTS

I guess most acknowledgements in books recognise the people who have helped bring the book to fruition. My acknowledgements are to thank the people who have kept me alive. This is an extensive list, and I have mentioned many of my supporters in the narrative.

Thank you to the healthcare professionals in Northampton General Hospital and Royal Derby Hospital, and to the scientists and researchers who are helping people like me to live a bit longer. A special thanks to Clare, my CNS.

A heartfelt thank you to all my family and friends. You have been, and continue to be, magnificent.

A few special mentions to pick out from the crowd:

Sally, my niece, who gave me hope, information and support.

Yvonne, my sister, who looked after me, thankfully, whether I wanted her to or not.

My partner, who has stuck with me through the good times and the bad.

My fabulous sons, Will and Dan, who are the best men I can imagine.

I am still alive because of you. xx

SOURCES OF HELP

targetovariancancer.org.uk

macmillan.org.uk

ovacome.org.uk

colostomyuk.org

AUTHOR PROFILE

Anita Gayton is a retired clinical psychologist. Leaving behind her varied career working with people with severe mental health problems, she enjoyed spending time with her adult sons, her partner and her family. She loved studying, travelling and keeping active, exercise sessions in the park and had just taken up walking football. She had always wanted to write a book. This was not the book she had in mind, but it was the book she felt she needed to write.

***

Thank you for purchasing this book. It means a lot that you have chosen to do so. I hope you found it a good read, although I realise it is not necessarily an easy read.

I would like as many people as possible to read it, as ovarian cancer is rarely talked about and I hope that sharing my story may help others. If you are able to spare a few minutes to post a review on Amazon, that would be much appreciated. It may encourage others to buy the book, and I will make a donation to an ovarian cancer charity for every book sold.

Publisher Information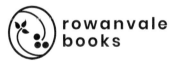

Rowanvale Books provides publishing services to independent authors, writers and poets all over the globe. We deliver a personal, honest and efficient service that allows authors to see their work published, while remaining in control of the process and retaining their creativity. By making publishing services available to authors in a cost-effective and ethical way, we at Rowanvale Books hope to ensure that the local, national and international community benefits from a steady stream of good quality literature.

For more information about us, our authors or our publications, please get in touch.

www.rowanvalebooks.com
info@rowanvalebooks.com

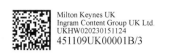

Milton Keynes UK
Ingram Content Group UK Ltd.
UKHW020230151124
451109UK00001B/3